INDIRA NANASHI OTOJ

HOW GUT BACTERIA CAN HELP YOU

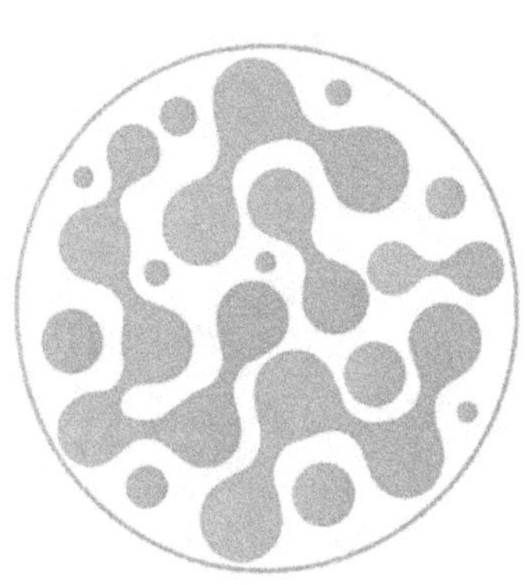

12 Problems Probiotics Can Solve

How Gut Bacteria Can Help You

12 Problems Probiotics Can Solve

Indira N. Otoj

Contents

Medical Disclaimer

The author is not an attorney, medical professional, nutritionist, mechanic, or dietitian. Content in this publication is for informational purposes only. It is not intended to substitute for legal or mechanical advice, or medical treatment or diagnosis. It is not monitored or evaluated by the Food and Drug Administration/FDA. Consult your health care provider if you are experiencing any symptoms and before using any supplement or biotic, or beginning a new health regimen. By using any or all of this information, you do so at your own risk. No warranties are expressed or implied. Any application of the material provided is at the reader's discretion and is his or her sole responsibility.

Introduction

I am not a gastroenterologist or an M.D. of any kind. So why am I writing this book, you ask? I am writing this book because I was intrigued from the moment I learned there were billions of tiny organisms living inside me. I was hooked on learning more about the concept of a "microbiome" and leveraging the little stowaways for my benefit however I could (or, at the very least, keep them from hurting me).

Probiotic, prebiotic, and to a lesser extent, the microbiome have become big buzzwords lately. Everybody sells a probiotic or prebiotic drink, pill, food, diet, or t-shirt. But what do these words even mean, and what do these 'biotics' do? And more importantly, what can they do and not do for *you*?

While considered a relatively new area of research, the study of the microbiome may go back further than you think. Humans have been curious about the gut for a long time but this interest was relegated mostly to the "oddballs" or "eccentrics" among us while the rest of us were happy to ignore our guts as long as everything worked properly.

Nobel laureate-microbiologist Joshua Lederberg coined the term microbiome in 2001, but the concept of microbes playing an instrumental role in biological (and ecological) systems dates back to the 1800s to Sergei Winogradsky, most likely, even earlier.

Even though the concept is old, we do not know a lot about the human microbiome and how it differs between individuals. We are also unaware of many of the effects various bacteria have on us and our gut.

However, research on the microbiome has increased in recent years. It has provided many insights into certain bacteria and bacterial families' function in and on our bodies. The National Institutes of Health (NIH) supported the Human Microbiome Project from 2007 to 2016, which contributed significantly to the body of research regarding the bacteria that live in and on the human body.

After achieving a basic understanding of the microbiome, researchers, mainly backed up by the

NIH, studied the connection between the microbiome and diseases and how to modify it to support health.

For example, in 2017, a review of 17 studies showed that giving probiotics to patients with antibiotics reduced by about half the likelihood of antibiotic-related diarrhea. In 2014, a systematic review of 21 students with ulcerative colitis showed that using probiotics can significantly improve the patients' overall health.[i] A review of 7 studies in 2018 showed that probiotics were an effective treatment for infant colic as well.

While research is ongoing, many peer-reviewed studies show that bacteria may be able to help us with the various ailments and issues we deal with every day.

So, what exactly *are* probiotics? Let's dive in.

What Are Probiotics?

Probiotics are live bacteria that are considered beneficial for your body, especially your digestive system. The term "probiotic" is often used to refer to supplements of good bacteria that can be ingested in food or pill form. Otherwise, the term gut biota, gut flora, or gut microbiome (or just microbiome for all bacteria in and on the body) is used to describe bacteria already present in a body. An imbalance in the gut flora is called dysbiosis and can lead to health issues large and small.

These good bacteria aim to keep your gut healthy by preventing the infiltration of bad bacteria and helping maintain various bodily functions. You can find several types of probiotics that can help in treating/preventing various bacterial infections and diseases. They also help your body digest well, create vitamins, and absorb medications. Let us look at the most common types of probiotics.

Lactobacilli

The most common probiotic is Lactobacillus (plural Lactobacilli but Lactobacillus will be used in the rest of this writing for recognizability), it is also known as Lactic Acid Bacteria (LAB) for reasons we will get into in a bit. It is taken orally for various digestive issues including diarrhea. It may also help with stomach pains, ulcerative colitis, eczema, allergies, vaginal infections, diabetes, and constipation. It is also used to improve mood and lower anxiety, control IBS, and promote weight loss.

Lactobacillus colonizes a person's body soon after birth, typically being introduced from the mother's vaginal canal and is a lifelong primary resident in our gut.

Lactobacillus produces lactic acid and acetate which are essential for balancing gut pH and encouraging the growth of other good bacteria. Acetate is a short chain fatty acid that feeds other bacteria in the gut that produce butyrate which is essential for a healthy gut lining. Lactobacillus also produces antimicrobial substances that help keep bad bacteria from colonizing the gut.

Lactobacillus is the most common probiotic found in pill form but is also found in many foods including yogurt, kefir, and other fermented foods. The Lactobacillus already in our gut can be further nourished with high fiber prebiotic foods (more on that later in the book).

Bifidobacteria

Another well-known probiotic family is Bifidobacterium. It lives in our intestines and stomach. Besides promoting a healthy gut, it may treat *Helicobacter pylori*, pouchitis, lung infections, and constipation.

According to a study in 2011, Bifidobacteria effectively improved global IBS symptoms with participants also reporting an improvement in their quality of life.[ii] It also may help in improving immunity by recruiting white blood cells to counter the effects of an infection.

Bifidobacteria are generally the first bacteria to colonize your gut. Like with Lactobacillus, this colonization process usually begins at birth with Bifidobacteria helping with milk digestion and immune system training. Bifidobacteria are lifelong helpers (similar to Lactobacillus) providing a host of other helpful if not essential functions including: breaking down and extracting nutrients from food we otherwise couldn't, producing B and K vitamins, balancing gut pH, and producing short chain fatty acids that feed other good bacteria.

Bifidobacteria can be found in many foods including vinegar, wines, cured meat, yogurt, and buttermilk.

Other types of probiotics

Common strains of probiotics include:

- *Lactobacillus acidophilus*
- *Lactobacillus plantarum*
- *Saccharomyces boulardii*
- *Bifidobacterium bifidum*
- *Bifidobacterium lactis*
- *Bifidobacterium longum*
- *Enterococcus faecium*
- *Lactobacillus bulgaricus*
- *Lactobacillus casei*
- *Lactobacillus gasseri*

FDA

Depending upon the use of a probiotic, the FDA may regulate it as a dietary supplement or a drug. Several probiotics are sold as nutritional supplements that do not need FDA approval. But manufacturers cannot make health claims without FDA approval.

To market a probiotic as a treatment for any disease, it must meet specific requirements, i.e., it should be proven effective *and* reliable through clinical testing and approved by the FDA.

The following chapters talk about different health complications people face, the causes, and how probiotics play a role in their treatment as well as possible side effects of probiotics.

12 Problems Probiotics Can Solve

Diarrhea

Bacterial diarrhea is often caused by Campylobacter, *Escherichia coli*, Salmonella, and Shigella bacteria. They enter your body through contaminated foods and drinks and infect the gastrointestinal tract.

However, probiotics can help you counter the effects of diarrhea, which may seem *very* counterintuitive at first. *Saccharomyces boulardii* is a type of yeast used as a probiotic and often marketed as a dietary supplement. According to studies, it works great against traveler's diarrhea and antibiotic-associated diarrhea and fights off unwanted pathogens such as *C. difficile* and *H. pylori*, both of which can cause diarrhea. [iii]

S. boulardii targets your gastrointestinal tract and helps restores bacterial balance, which is disturbed by infectious bacteria. It is commonly found in mangosteen and lychee fruits. It is also available in pill and powder forms.

IBS and Gut Infections

Irritable bowel syndrome, commonly known as IBS, is sometimes developed after experiencing diarrhea caused by a bacterial infection. Bacterial overgrowth in the intestines may also cause it. IBS causes severe abdominal pain, bloating, gas, and cramping. Some of the intestinal bacteria that play a role in this are *Clostridium perfringens*, Staphylococcus bacteria, and *E. coli*.

Probiotics have been suggested to reduce visceral hypersensitivity and exert anti-inflammatory effects. However, the results vary for each person. [iv]

For example, a probiotic, *Lactobacillus Plantarum 299V*, was studied in about 112 patients. Symptoms like pain and gas improved, but there was a negligible improvement in constipation.

Another study that included *Streptococcus thermophilus, Lactobacillus bulgaricus*, and

Bifidobacterium longum had a comparatively better result, further improving the symptoms of IBS.

These probiotics are found in fermented foods like sourdough, pickles, and yogurt.

Constipation

Constipation is the most common gastrointestinal complaint in the USA. At least 2.5 million people are seen by doctors each year for constipation. Symptoms of constipation include dry, lumpy stools, stomach ache and cramps, bloating and nausea, and difficult or painful passing of stool.

Constipation can be an ongoing, annoying and, more rarely, serious affliction if it causes hemorrhoids, anal fissures, diverticulitis, or incontinence. There are potential treatments beyond laxatives however.

Probiotics, especially when paired with prebiotics (more on them later) have been shown to be effective in combating constipation. Particularly, the strains *Bifidobacterium lactis* and *B. longum* have been shown to work quite well.

Bifidobacteria can be found in fermented foods as well as yogurt and can often be found in pill form.

Stress, Anxiety and Depression

Stress, anxiety, and depression are often interrelated. Recent studies have shown that the bacteria present in the gut help regulate brain functions through the gut-brain axis. One implication of this is that what you eat really can affect your mood.

The GBA links the brain's emotional and cognitive centers with the gut; therefore, the gut microbiota plays a vital role in regulating mood, sleep patterns, and resilience.

Stress and anxiety can cause changes in the types and number of bacteria in the gut (the reverse may also be true). Even though the communication between the brain and the gut is bidirectional, it appears the connection from the gut to the brain is stronger than the brain to the gut. This means that gut changes can have a stronger effect on your brain than previously thought possible, and your brain does not heavily regulate your gut.

Probiotics formulations of *L. helveticus* R0052 and *B. longum* R0175A were observed to reduce stress and anxiety in humans and rats.[v]

However, the *L. rhamnosus* strain has the most evidence showcasing that it can significantly reduce anxiety.

Fermented foods such as kraut, kimchi, and yogurt often contain not only Lactobacillus but also Bifidobacteria.

Dementia

According to recent studies, Alzheimer's, a common form of dementia, is possibly due to an infection caused by the bacteria Porphyromonas gingivalis. It releases toxins known as gingipains that target proteins that over time can have a drastic effect on the brain. [vi]

Signs of dementia can be difficult to see at first but can get gradually worse with time. A person can forget to pay bills or have trouble remembering appointments. The damage done to brain cells due to this disease interferes with cell communication.

According to a study by <u>Chyn Boon Wong</u>, *"Increasing evidence from preclinical and clinical studies has demonstrated that probiotics possess preventive as well as the therapeutic potential for AD."* [vii]

Lactobacillus and Bifidobacteria are believed to improve the patient's condition moderately, but research is still ongoing. Testing on mice has shown that probiotics have aided in their learning and memory.

A <u>study</u> in Kashan University of Medical Sciences and Islamic Azad University in Iran conducted tests on two groups of people. The probiotics used in the study included *L. acidophilus*, *L. casei*, *L. fermentum*, and *B. bifidum*. One group was given milk with these probiotics, and the other group was given plain milk daily for about 12 weeks. The group that was given the probiotics had significantly better test scores. [viii]

Weight Changes

Gut bacteria come directly in contact with your food. Therefore, it significantly affects the nutrients absorbed and storage of energy.

In one twin study, where one twin was obese and the other of normal weight, the twins' gut bacteria were noted to be different. In the obese twin, there was lower gut bacteria diversity.[ix]

The two bacteria that have been shown to heavily influence weight are Prevotella (digests fiber and carbohydrates) and Bacteroidetes, which is present mostly in people who consume more animal protein.

Akkermansia muciniphila and *Christensenella minuta* are considered 'good bacteria' and prevent unhealthy weight gain. You can easily find these in everyday foods such as cranberries, black tea, flax seeds, and bamboo shoots.

Bloating

Bloating is a common symptom of small intestinal bacterial overgrowth (SIBO). It can also be caused due to eating or drinking too quickly, smoking, or wearing loose dentures. Other medical reasons can be weight gain, irritable bowel syndrome, and heartburn.

Bilophila wadsworthia is a bacterium that produces hydrogen sulfide gas, which results in irritation, bloating, and gas.

In a study, a probiotic containing *L. casei, L. plantarum, Streptococcus faecalis*, and *B. brevis* was suggested to improve the overall condition of patients with SIBO.[x]

Other than SIBO, bloating and stomach pain is also a common symptom of lactose intolerance. It is a disorder where the body does not digest lactose due to the lack of the enzyme, lactase.

The colon breaks down the undigested lactose that releases gases like carbon dioxide, methane, and hydrogen.

One study showed the probiotic strain of *L. acidophilus* can improve abdominal symptoms of those suffering from lactose intolerance.[xi]

Bacterial Vaginosis (BV)

Bacterial vaginosis is a common type of bacterial infection among women where the pH of the vagina is disrupted. It is usually indicated through a thin yellow/grey discharge, which has a strong smell. This infection is usually a result of the overgrowth of *Gardnerella Vaginalis* bacteria.[xii]

G. Vaginalis is a healthy bacterium that is also the most common type of bacteria in the vagina. But the growth of this bacteria in excess can lead to infection. This can have varying causes such as douching, using vaginal deodorants, other irritating products, and unprotected sex. BV can also increase the risk of contracting an STD.

Probiotics can be beneficial in the treatment of BV. *L. acidophilus* may help to prevent this type of infection. *L. acidophilus* can be commonly found in yogurt and other dairy products, the ingestion of which may ease some of the symptoms associated with infection or reduce the chances of infection or reoccurrence. [xvii]

Helicobacter pylori

H. pylori lives in the digestive tract of as many as half of the people on the planet and can cause ulcers in the lining of the stomach. As it enters the body, it targets the stomach lining and damages it. The acid that your body uses to digest food can get through the lining and create ulcers. *H. pylori* infection can also lead to stomach cancer. However, most people who have *H. pylori* in their gut will never know as they will never experience negative side effects.

Although many people do not experience any symptoms from having *H. pylori*, some can experience nausea, loss of appetite, and bloating with black stool and severe abdominal pain requiring immediate medical attention. *H. pylori* can be transmitted through direct contact with saliva, vomit, and fecal matter, or through contaminated food and water. Living in a place with many people or without a clean water source can increase your risk of contracting *H. pylori*.

Probiotics such as Lactobacillus and Bifidobacteria can reduce the negative side effects of *H. pylori* and decrease the amount found in the gut. [xiii]

Urinary Tract Infection (UTI)

Any infection in any part of your urinary system is known as an urinary tract infection. It is more likely to occur in women than in men. Some common symptoms can be pain in the pelvic region, urine that appears to be cloudy, and a burning sensation when passing urine.

Infections frequently occur in the bladder or urethra. They are often caused by *E. coli*, which lives in the digestive tract. Apart from *E. coli*, Staphylococcus can also contribute to an infection.

Lactobacillus is observed to counter the effects of *E. coli* and prevent its growth. In one study, probiotic capsules containing *L. fermentes* and *L. rhamnosus* were observed to have a significant role in preventing UTIs. [xiv]

Prebiotics

Prebiotics, another big buzzword. But what are they? Generally, prebiotics are carbs your body can't digest i.e., fiber. Prebiotics are like food for your gut bacteria.

Many foods contain prebiotics (aka various types of fiber) such as oats and other whole grains, fruits such as bananas and berries, and vegetables such as garlic and asparagus. The foods listed here are particularly good for helping Bifidobacteria thrive. Foods containing polyphenols such as green tea, cocoa, and red wine have also been shown to increase the amount of Bifidobacteria in the gut. [xv][xvi]

Other prebiotic foods include Konjac flour, soy, barley, walnuts, chokeberry, apples, artichoke, and chicory root. All of which are good for maintaining Lactobacillus levels.

Common Side Effects of Probiotics

Even though probiotics have shown remarkable results in many studies, a few studies have suggested that they may lead to unpleasant side effects. There is also a greater risk of probiotics harming individuals with weak or compromised immune systems.

Effects vary in severity, including infections, production of harmful substances, and transfer of antibiotic resistance traits from the good bacteria to the harmful bacteria in the digestive tract. Probiotics are notorious for helping alleviate and at the same time potentially exacerbating certain conditions depending on the specific strain used and other factors…

Constipation

Common side effects of some probiotics include gas and bloating. Moreover, yeast-based probiotics can result in individuals experiencing constipation. It is still somewhat unclear as to why this happens. To prevent this, it is recommended to go slowly and increase a probiotic dosage over a few weeks to give your body time to adjust to any new probiotic regimen.

Headaches

Fermented foods contain biogenic amines. They cause headaches as they activate the nervous system and alter the blood flow. However, this varies for each individual, and research is still needed to determine whether biogenic amines actually cause headaches. A good alternative to foods containing probiotics would be a probiotic supplement.

Allergic Reactions

Probiotic strains can produce histamines inside your body. Histamine is a molecule produced by your immune system when a threat is detected. When its level rises, blood vessels dilate, which results in swelling and allergic reactions. When this is present in excess and not properly degraded, it can result in an allergic reaction. Therefore, those with a histamine intolerance should avoid probiotic strains such as *L.*

hilgardii, *L. buchneri*, *L. helveticus*, and *Streptococcus thermophiles*.

Lactose Intolerance

Some probiotic supplements also include ingredients that may cause allergies, like dairy, soy, milk, and egg. Even though lactose intolerant individuals may be able to consume up to 400 mg of lactose, a few have noticed adverse effects. Therefore, those with lactose intolerance should choose lactose-free products to avoid complications.

Gas Bloating

Prebiotics are also present in some probiotic products. Side effects of prebiotics especially include gas and bloating although probiotics may cause these symptoms as well. Gas and bloating typically subside with the continued use of a probiotic.

Infections

Some cases have been reported that bacteria or yeast in probiotics could seep into the bloodstream and cause infections. The ones who are at the greatest risk of this are those with compromised immune systems and who have undergone recent surgeries. However, the risk is very low, estimated at less than one in one million for lactobacilli products.

Summary

Bacteria:	Use:
Saccharomyces boulardii	Treat diarrhea
Streptococcus thermophilus, Lactobacillus bulgaricus, L. plantarum and *Bifidobacterium longum*	Prevention and management of IBS symptoms
B. lactis and **B. longum**	Combat constipation
L. helveticus and **B. longum** , and **L.** *rhamnosus*	Improve symptoms of anxiety and depression
L. acidophilus, L. casei, L. fermentum, and **B. bifidum**	Improve memory; may help protect from dementia and Alzheimer's
Prevotella, *Akkermansia muciniphila* and **Christensenella minuta**	May help encourage weight loss
L. casei, L. plantarum, Streptococcus faecalis, and **B. brevis**	Reduce bloating and help combat small intestinal bacterial overgrowth (SIBO)
L. acidophilus	Reduce symptoms of lactose intolerance Help treat bacterial vaginosis
Lactobacillus spp. and **Bifidobacterium spp.**	Help treat *H. pylori* infection
L. fermentes and **L. rhamnosus**	Help prevent UTIs

Conclusion

Bacteria play a vital role in helping us maintain healthy body functions, from helping with digestion, producing vitamins, and regulating our weight to helping maintain healthy blood sugar levels, regulating our immune system, and affecting our mood. If used the right way, probiotics (whether in food or pill form) can be an effective solution against a bevy of infections and diseases too!

Every day, researchers are looking for and finding more beneficial uses for bacteria and discovering more about what and how the bacteria already in our bodies affect us. The old school belief that all bacteria is bad and must be destroyed is being scrubbed from modern thought.

References

---

[i] Ghouri, Y. A., Richards, D. M., Rahimi, E. F., Krill, J. T., Jelinek, K. A., & DuPont, A. W. (2014). Systematic review of randomized controlled trials of probiotics, prebiotics, and symbiotics in inflammatory bowel disease. *Clinical and experimental gastroenterology, 7*, 473–487. https://doi.org/10.2147/CEG.S27530

[ii] Guglielmetti, S., Mora, D., Gschwender, M., & Popp, K. (2011). Randomised clinical trial: Bifidobacterium bifidum MIMBb75 significantly alleviates irritable bowel syndrome and improves quality of life--a double-blind, placebo-controlled study. *Alimentary pharmacology & therapeutics, 33*(10), 1123–1132. https://doi.org/10.1111/j.1365-2036.2011.04633.x

[iii] Kelesidis, T., & Pothoulakis, C. (2012). Efficacy and safety of the probiotic Saccharomyces boulardii for the prevention and therapy of gastrointestinal disorders. *Therapeutic advances in gastroenterology, 5*(2), 111–125. https://doi.org/10.1177/1756283X11428502

[iv] Menees, S., & Chey, W. (2018). The gut microbiome and irritable bowel syndrome. *F1000Research, 7*, F1000 Faculty Rev-1029. https://doi.org/10.12688/f1000research.14592.1

[v] Irvine, E. J. (2004). Patients' fears and unmet needs in inflammatory bowel disease. *Alimentary pharmacology & therapeutics, 20*, 54-59.

[vi] Dominy, S. S., Lynch, C., Ermini, F., Benedyk, M., Marczyk, A., Konradi, A., Nguyen, M., Haditsch, U., Raha, D., Griffin, C., Holsinger, L. J., Arastu-Kapur, S., Kaba, S., Lee, A., Ryder, M. I., Potempa, B., Mydel, P., Hellvard, A., Adamowicz, K., Hasturk, H., … Potempa, J. (2019). *Porphyromonas gingivalis* in Alzheimer's disease

brains: Evidence for disease causation and treatment with small-molecule inhibitors. *Science advances*, 5(1), eaau3333. https://doi.org/10.1126/sciadv.aau3333

[vii] Wong, C. B., Kobayashi, Y., & Xiao, J. Z. (2018). Probiotics for preventing cognitive impairment in Alzheimer's disease. *Gut Microbiota-Brain Axis*, 85-104.

[viii] Akbari E, Asemi Z, Daneshvar Kakhaki R, et al. Effect of probiotic supplementation on cognitive function and metabolic status in Alzheimer's disease: a randomized, double-blind, and controlled trial. Front Aging Neurosci. 2016; 8:256. doi: 10.3389/fnagi.2016.00256.

[ix] Ridaura, V. K., Faith, J. J., Rey, F. E., Cheng, J., Duncan, A. E., Kau, A. L., Griffin, N. W., Lombard, V., Henrissat, B., Bain, J. R., Muehlbauer, M. J., Ilkayeva, O., Semenkovich, C. F., Funai, K., Hayashi, D. K., Lyle, B. J., Martini, M. C., Ursell, L. K., Clemente, J. C., Van Treuren, W., ... Gordon, J. I. (2013). Gut microbiota from twins discordant for obesity modulate metabolism in mice. *Science (New York, N.Y.)*, *341*(6150), 1241214. https://doi.org/10.1126/science.1241214

[x] Soifer, L. O., Peralta, D., Dima, G., & Besasso, H. (2010). Eficacia comparativa de un probiótico vs un antibiótico en la respuesta clínica de pacientes con sobrecrecimiento bacteriano del intestino y distensión abdominal crónica funcional: un estudio piloto [Comparative clinical efficacy of a probiotic vs. an antibiotic in the treatment of patients with intestinal bacterial overgrowth and chronic abdominal functional distension: a pilot study]. *Acta gastroenterologica Latinoamericana, 40*(4), 323–327.

[xi] Pakdaman, M.N., Udani, J.K., Molina, J.P. *et al.* The effects of the DDS-1 strain of lactobacillus on symptomatic relief for lactose intolerance - a randomized, double-blind,

placebo-controlled, crossover clinical trial. *Nutr J* **15**, 56 (2015). https://doi.org/10.1186/s12937-016-0172-y

[xii] : Cribby, S., Taylor, M., & Reid, G. (2008). Vaginal microbiota and the use of probiotics. *Interdisciplinary perspectives on infectious diseases, 2008*, 256490. https://doi.org/10.1155/2008/256490

[xiii] Homan, M., & Orel, R. (2015). Are probiotics useful in Helicobacter pylori eradication? *World journal of gastroenterology, 21*(37), 10644–10653. https://doi.org/10.3748/wjg.v21.i37.10644

[xiv] Akgül, T., & Karakan, T. (2018). The role of probiotics in women with recurrent urinary tract infections. *Turkish journal of urology, 44*(5), 377–383. https://doi.org/10.5152/tud.2018.48742

[xv] Queipo-Ortuño MI, Boto-Ordóñez M, Murri M, Gomez-Zumaquero JM, Clemente-Postigo M, Estruch R, Cardona Diaz F, Andrés-Lacueva C, Tinahones FJ. Influence of red wine polyphenols and ethanol on the gut microbiota ecology and biochemical biomarkers. Am J Clin Nutr. 2012 Jun;95(6):1323-34. doi: 10.3945/ajcn.111.027847. Epub 2012 May 2. PMID: 22552027.

[xvi] Tzounis X, Rodriguez-Mateos A, Vulevic J, Gibson GR, Kwik-Uribe C, Spencer JP. Prebiotic evaluation of cocoa-derived flavanols in healthy humans by using a randomized, controlled, double-blind, crossover intervention study. Am J Clin Nutr. 2011 Jan;93(1):62-72. doi: 10.3945/ajcn.110.000075. Epub 2010 Nov 10. PMID: 21068351.

[xvii] Falagas, M., Betsi, G. I., & Athanasiou, S. (2007). Probiotics for the treatment of women with bacterial vaginosis. *Clinical microbiology and infection : the official publication of the European Society of Clinical Microbiology and Infectious Diseases, 13*(7), 657–664. https://doi.org/10.1111/j.1469-0691.2007.01688.x

[xviii] Doeun, D., Davaatseren, M., & Chung, M. S. (2017).

Biogenic amines in foods. *Food science and biotechnology, 26*(6), 1463–1474. https://doi.org/10.1007/s10068-017-0239-3

www.ingramcontent.com/pod-product-compliance
Lightning Source LLC
Chambersburg PA
CBHW061325250726
48657CB00003B/1049